Dr. Andrew Weil is the leader in the new field of Integrative Medicine, which combines the best ideas and practices of conventional and alternative medicine. A graduate of Harvard Medical School, he is director of the Program in Integrative Medicine at the University of Arizona, the first program to train physicians in this way at an American medical school. He is also the founder of the Center for Integrative Medicine in Tucson, which is advancing the field worldwide. Dr. Weil is well known as an expert in natural medicine, mind-body interactions, and medical botany, as well as the author of the best-selling *Spontaneous Healing* and *8 Weeks to Optimum Health*. According to Dr. Weil, 'Spontaneous healing is not a miracle or a lucky exception, but a fact of biology, the result of the natural healing system that each of us is born with.'

The 'Ask Dr. Weil' program (www.drweil.com) features Andrew Weil, M.D., and is one of the top-rated health sites on the World Wide Web and is featured on Time Warner's Pathfinder Network. The recipient of many awards, it features a daily Q&A with answers to a wide range of health questions, a daily poll, and the Doc Weil Database, which lets readers search hundreds of topics, including material from Dr. Weil's bestselling book *Natural Health, Natural Medicine*. The site also features a Referral Directory (practitioners from acupuncture to Trager work) and DocTalk, a live weekly chat with Dr. Weil. If you have additional questions for Dr. Weil, ask them on his Web site.

D1103063

By Andrew Weil, M.D.:

Ask Dr. Weil
WOMEN'S HEALTH
YOUR TOP HEALTH CONCERNS
NATURAL REMEDIES
VITAMINS AND MINERALS
COMMON ILLNESSES
HEALTHY LIVING

8 WEEKS TO OPTIMUM HEALTH
SPONTANEOUS HEALING
NATURAL HEALTH, NATURAL MEDICINE
HEALTH AND HEALING
FROM CHOCOLATE TO MORPHINE
THE MARRIAGE OF THE SUN AND THE MOON
THE NATURAL MIND

Ask Dr. Weil

Women's Health

Andrew Weil, M.D.
Edited by Steven Petrow

WARNER BOOKS

Questions contained in this book may appear in other volumes of the *Ask Dr. Weil* series. The books are arranged according to topic, and to create a complete health profile utilizing Dr. Weil's prescriptions, material may overlap.

A *Warner* Book

First published in Great Britain in 1998 by Warner Books

Published in the United States by Ballantine Books, a division of Random House, Inc., New York 1997

Copyright © Great Bear Productions, LLC 1997

This work was compiled from the *Ask Dr. Weil* Web Site.

The moral right of the author has been asserted.

A CIP catalogue record for this book is available from the British Library

ISBN 0 7515 2607 x

Typeset in Berkeley by M Rules
Printed and bound in Great Britain by Clays Ltd, St Ives plc

Warner Books
A Division of
Little, Brown and Company (UK)
Brettenham House
Lancaster Place
London WC2E 7EN

Introduction

You've taken the first step toward optimum health. This book will give you more information about my philosophy along with answers to some of the questions I am asked most frequently.

I wrote *Spontaneous Healing* and *8 Weeks to Optimum Health* because I wanted to call attention to the innate, intrinsic nature of the healing process. I've always believed that the body can heal itself if you give it a chance. Why? Because it has a healing system. If you're feeling well, it's important to know about this system so that you can enhance your well-being. If you are ill, you'll also want to know about it because it is your best hope of recovery.

To maintain optimum health requires commitment. This book – and the others in the series – can give you much of the basic information you need about diet, supplements, common illnesses, natural remedies, and healthy living.

All of these questions originated on 'Ask Dr. Weil', my program on the World Wide Web. If you still have questions, come visit the clinic at www.drweil.com.

Can Animal Hormones Harm Kids?

Q:

A friend told me her nine-year-old daughter already has had her first period, as have most of her classmates! She says it's because of the estrogen they consume from additives in dairy and beef. Is this true? Are these girls typical?

A:

You're correct that the onset of menstruation has been getting progressively earlier among girls in the United States. No one is sure why, but one possibility is that commercially produced meat and milk products contain residues of growth-promoting hormones. These have estrogenic activity, so they could stimulate early menstruation.

Some years ago, there was an epidemic of premature puberty in very young girls (under four years old) in Puerto Rico. This was traced to consumption of chicken carrying unusually high residues of estrogenic hormones.

Another disturbing possibility is that many environmental pollutants, including some pesticides and plastics, may act like estrogens in the body. Eating soy foods may offer protection from them.

There's reason to be concerned about early onset of menstruation, because it's a factor of significant risk for breast cancer. Women who menstruate early will have more years of exposure to their own estrogens, which stimulate the cells of the breasts and reproductive system to proliferate.

I would minimize the amount of animal food fed to children, or use only organically produced meat, poultry, or dairy products certified to be free of hormones. And try to get the kids to eat tofu!

What Is Your
Antioxidant Cocktail?

Q:
What vitamins should I be taking on a regular basis?

A:
I get asked about the antioxidant 'cocktail' perhaps more than about any other subject. You can really help your body by taking protective antioxidants, nutrients that protect tissues by blocking the chemical reactions by which many toxins cause harm. One way to go about it is to increase your consumption of fresh fruits and vegetables. You can also take supplements.

Here is the formula I use myself and recommend to my patients:

- *Vitamin C:* 1,000 to 2,000 milligrams two to three times a day. Your body can absorb this vitamin more easily in a soluble powder form than in a large tablet. I take a dose of vitamin C with breakfast and dinner, and, if I can remember, another before bed. Plain ascorbic acid may irritate a sensitive stomach, so take it with food or look for a buffered or nonacidic form.
- *Vitamin E:* 400 to 800 IU a day. People under forty should take 400 IU a day; people over forty, 800 IU.

Since vitamin E is fat soluble, it must be taken with food to be absorbed. Also, natural vitamin E (d-alpha-tocopherol) is much better than the synthetic form (dl-alpha-tocopherol). I usually take vitamin E at lunch. Make sure the product contains the other tocopherols, especially gamma, which offers protection that alphatocopherol does not.

- *Selenium:* 200 to 300 micrograms a day. Selenium is a trace mineral with antioxidant and anticancer properties. Selenium and vitamin E facilitate each other's absorption, so take them together. Vitamin C may interfere with the absorption of some forms of selenium, so take them separately. Doses above 400 micrograms a day may not be healthy.

- *Mixed carotenes:* 25,000 IU a day. I take mixed carotenes as a supplement with my breakfast. I recommend a natural form – easily found in health food stores. Men: read the label to make sure it gives you lycopene, the red pigment in tomatoes that helps prevent prostate cancer.

All in all, this is a simple formula that will not cost you too much trouble or money.

Natural Methods of
Birth Control?

Q:

I have been on the Pill for eight years. I'm tired of the mood swings, the increase in yeast infections, etc. A close friend uses a natural method that involves the monitoring of vaginal discharge together with an awareness of stages of her cycle, and she manages to avoid having intercourse during ovulation time. I have decided – with my husband's agreement – to try this. Do you know anything about this natural method?

A:

I think it's a good idea to go off the Pill if you can find other ways to practice contraception. The current generation of oral contraceptives are safer than those of the past, because they use lower doses of hormones. But you are still exposing the body to the very general effects of hormones, rather than getting just the specific effect on fertility that you desire. High levels of female sex hormones favor the development of cancer of the breast and of the reproductive system. And while there aren't any data clearly linking oral contraceptives to a higher risk of cancer, there is reason for caution.

Oral contraceptives also increase the risk of blood clots, and many women experience side effects such as nausea, breast tenderness, fluid retention, weight gain, and depression. The Pill reduces interest in sex over time, although triphasic versions, which vary the amount of synthetic progesterone and estrogen over the month, have less of this effect. If you smoke, have a family history of breast cancer, have a history of benign breast disease, did not have a first child until after age thirty-five, are over forty-five and still menstruating, or are at increased risk of cervical cancer because of multiple sex partners, I'd definitely say stay off the Pill.

If a woman becomes very aware of her body's cycles and pays attention to things like her temperature and the texture of her cervical mucus, I think it's possible for her to rely on a natural method. Certainly there are advantages, because a lot of women can't tolerate the side effects of the Pill.

You do need to recognize, however, that the natural method is less reliable and requires conscientious effort by both partners. The calendar rhythm method is least reliable. Measuring the woman's basal body temperature each morning is more accurate, as is watching for changes in the texture and amount of cervical mucus. A combination of these techniques is the most effective, but even with training in ways to monitor ovulation, the failure rate is still about 10 per cent a year. Tracking ovulation is easier for some women than others, depending on the nature of their cycle.

But the natural method isn't the only way to go if you decide not to take the Pill. You can also choose condoms, foam and condoms, a contraceptive sponge, a diaphragm, or a cervical cap, which is similar to a diaphragm but can be left in the vagina longer.

Lower Your Risk for Breast Cancer?

Q:
What specific things can women do to reduce the risk of breast cancer? It's well-publicized that early breast-feeding is helpful. Can you give specific dietary recommendations or other suggestions? Thanks.

A:
Breast cancer results from a complex interaction of genetic and environmental factors. While we do not know all the details of its origin, we can make specific recommendations for lifestyle changes that will reduce risk. Some of these are intended to reduce estrogen production in the body or limit exposure to foreign estrogens. Those hormones stimulate breast cells to grow and divide, increasing the chance of malignant transformation. Other recommendations are aimed at strengthening the body's defenses.

Women who begin menstruating early have a higher risk of breast cancer, as do those who reach menopause late. Such women are exposed to estrogen for longer periods of time. Having a first baby at a younger age and breast-feeding both lessen the risk of breast cancer, probably by interrupting the menstrual cycle and reducing lifetime estrogen exposure. You may not be able to change much here, but you can make choices about your diet that will affect the amount of estrogen in your body.

Animal fats contribute to increased estrogen levels in the body, and a low-fat diet has been shown to help guard against breast cancer. Commercially raised animal foods often contain residues of estrogenic hormones given to animals as growth promoters. If you are a carnivore, you should contact the Soil Association (see Other Resources on p. 86) for sources of organic meat.

Soy products such as tofu, tempeh, and miso, which are full of weak, plant-based estrogens, lower cancer risk, perhaps because they occupy estrogen receptors, protecting them from stronger forms of the hormone (such as many environmental pollutants). Compounds in cabbage block stronger surges of estrogen from other sources. A chemical in cabbage, broccoli, and kale, also may be helpful.

On the other hand, alcohol, even in moderate usage, can increase estrogen production in susceptible women.

Regular, moderate exercise – four hours a week – reduced breast cancer risk before menopause by an average of 58 per cent in one study. Researchers believe it lowers estrogen production. After menopause, exercise may still help by lessening body fat, another factor in estrogen exposure.

So the most important thing to think about is protecting the overall health and well-being of your body. Exercise regularly. Minimize your exposure to environmental estrogenic pollutants by eating low on the food chain. Especially limit your intake of commercially raised meats, dairy products, and eggs. Eat lots of fruits, vegetables, and soy foods and plenty of fiber to keep estrogen levels under control and protect your genes from damage. Also, take antioxidants to guard against deleterious mutations and protect immune defenses.

If you know you're at high risk, take two tablespoons of ground linseed on your cereal or in your juice every day. Linseed reduces the rate of growth of tumors in rats and lowers the chance of cancers getting started in the first place.

Finally, note that the role of psychological factors in breast cancer is not at all clear. Grief and depression may suppress immunity, allowing cancers to grow faster. But I doubt that they play much of a role in their origin. Women with this disease did not 'give themselves cancer' as a result of any sort of emotional failure.

How to Treat Chlamydia?

Q:

A woman claims to have picked up chlamydia from me twice, in 1986 and 1989. I couldn't have given it to her, since I never had any symptoms. Pelvic inflammatory disease was diagnosed in her in 1986 and chlamydia in 1989. Tetracycline was prescribed to her both times. No M.D. ever asked to speak to me. Doctors have told me that chlamydia testing was extremely unreliable back then and as recently as 1992 was stopped at George Washington Medical Center because of high false positives and negatives. Is there any way to test now if I ever had it? Is there any record of test reliability in that time period? Would I have any noticeable symptoms if I had it? Any other comments?

A:

Chlamydia is the most common sexually transmitted disease, with an estimated 4 million infections from the organism occurring every year. The infection can cause serious problems in women, beginning with pelvic inflammatory disease and possibly leading to ectopic pregnancy or infertility. Almost three-quarters of women with the disease don't notice any symptoms, which can include vaginal discharge or painful urination.

Diagnosis of chlamydia is difficult, as you point out, but some newer and more accurate diagnostic tests are available. Scientists at Johns Hopkins have developed a new urine test for chlamydia that is simpler, more convenient, and just as sensitive as older methods (taking small scrapings of cells from a woman's cervix or a swab from a man's urethra). The Hopkins test uses a technology called DNA amplification, which is like a super-copying machine for genes. By producing millions of copies of genetic material found in the *Chlamydia* organism, this test makes the disease more easily detectable in the laboratory. The Hopkins test is especially useful to determine if treatment has been successful.

There's certainly no way to test now whether you had it years ago. There's a high chance that chlamydia will be asymptomatic in men, which is one of the reasons it gets passed around so much. In fact, reported cases for women are more than five times as great as for men, in part because men are rarely tested for it.

When the symptoms do occur in men, they commonly include mildly painful urination and a scanty to moderate penile discharge. You probably should have received tetracycline in the same dose as your partner. Anytime one sex partner has chlamydia, the other one should be treated as well.

Finally, I think it's important to remember that both parties need to take responsibility for sexual health these days. I detect a tone in your question, implying that your woman friend was somehow at fault. Laying blame has no place in this discussion.

Help for Chronic Fatigue Syndrome?

Q:

My wife has had chronic fatigue syndrome for the past six years. Traditional medicine has seemed to offer very little and in the past has actually made her worse. Many M.D.s, including many who specialize in the field, still seem not to have a clue about how to treat this illness. What suggestions do you have for overcoming this disease?

A:

Many people have written in to my Web program about chronic fatigue syndrome (CFS), a condition known incorrectly as 'chronic Epstein-Barr virus disease' or 'chronic EBV'. I'm not sure anybody knows exactly what chronic fatigue syndrome is; right now it appears to be a faddish disease that may or may not prove to be a true clinical entity. My suspicion is that if you look at a hundred people with the diagnosis, you might actually find many different conditions present – some purely emotional (such as depression) and others that might involve chronic viral infections.

The most important information I can give you is that the syndrome will end. Don't believe people who tell you otherwise.

I agree that conventional medicine has little to offer. Some doctors attempt treatment with injections of gamma globulin, interferon, or the antiviral drug acyclovir. These are pretty drastic methods that may do more harm than good. It sounds as though your wife has already been subjected to some of these treatments; generally I advise staying away from them.

Unfortunately, alternative practitioners often take advantage of patients with CFS and charge them a lot of money for treatments of questionable value. Here are my general recommendations for people with CFS:

- Take astragalus root for its antiviral and immunity-enhancing properties. I've used a U.S. product called Astra-8, a mixture of astragalus and seven other Chinese herbs. Take three tablets twice a day. You should have no problem staying on it indefinitely.
- Take maitake mushrooms, generally available in health food stores. These are nontoxic and may speed recovery. Follow dosages on the product container.
- Take my antioxidant formula (see page 3). In addition, take 60–100 milligrams of coenzyme Q, plus a B-100 B-complex supplement.
- Eat a low-protein, low-fat, high-carbohydrate diet.
- Eat one to two cloves of raw garlic a day. Garlic is a potent antibiotic, with antibacterial and antiviral effects as well. (By the way, a clove of garlic is one of the segments making up the head or bulb. Don't eat the whole bulb!) Chop it fine and mix with food, or swallow chunks like pills.
- Be careful about joining support groups. Find a group

that encourages recovery, not the idea that you will be sick forever.

Again, tell your wife not to despair. Many of my patients have recovered. I'd like to hear back from you in two to three months, after you've tried these methods.

Cursing Your Cramps?

Q:
Is there any way to stop cramps while having my period – other than with painkillers?

A:
Two-thirds of all women suffer from menstrual cramps. Until a couple of decades ago, the pain they endured was written off as a psychological 'female problem' that women created for themselves. But in the late 1970s, researchers discovered a hormone called prostaglandin F_2 alpha that is released as the uterine lining breaks down, causing the uterus to go into spasm and hurt.

You can moderate the release of PGF_2 alpha through some dietary measures, primarily a low-fat, high-complex carbohydrate diet. Don't eat dairy products, and lessen up on the meat and eggs. Cut back on fried foods and commercially baked foods. Most important, make sure you get enough essential fatty acids. If you have plenty of essential fatty acids in your system, your body will produce less PGF_2 alpha and more of a different hormone that helps prevent cramps. In one study, women who took 1.8 grams of omega-3 fatty acids in fish-oil capsules twice a day for two months had a significant improvement in cramps, nausea, and headaches. They used half as much aspirin as they had previously. I know other women who say oil of evening primrose works wonderfully for the same purpose, at a dose of two to three 500-milligram capsules twice a day.

In *Women's Bodies, Women's Wisdom*, Christiane Northrup, M.D., recommends a series of supplements to protect against cramps: 100 milligrams of vitamin B-6 per day, 50 IU of vitamin E (in the form of d-alpha tocopherol) three times a day, and 100 milligrams of magnesium three to four times a day. While you're menstruating, she suggests as much as 100 milligrams of magnesium every two hours to ease pain.

There are some effective traditional remedies for cramps as well, such as raspberry leaf tea. It's nontoxic, so you can consume as much as you like. An herb called cramp bark (*Viburnum opulus*), from a European bush, is a stronger remedy. The dose is one dropperful of the tincture in warm water as needed.

I'd also try acupuncture. There are pressure points that some people say will help, such as the acupuncture point on the wrist that's used for alleviating nausea, or a point on the inside of the foot that's used by reflexologists.

Smoking has been linked to added menstrual pain. And remember how much an influence stress can be. Try to reduce stress in your life and practice relaxation techniques, such as meditation or yoga.

For added relief, you can put a hot water bottle over your abdomen. And try massaging in a menstrual cramp oil recommended by Kathi Keville in *Herbs for Health and Healing*:

2 ounces Saint-John's-wort oil

8 drops each lavender, marjoram, and chamomile essential oils

Combine ingredients and use for any kind of muscle cramps.

Does Deodorant
Cause Breast Cancer?

Q:

Given that the sweat glands of the armpits are in close proximity to the breasts, has any research ever been done to see whether the use of deodorants has a positive correlation to the incidence of breast cancer in women?

A:

I'm not aware of any research on that topic. However, deodorants containing antiperspirants commonly cause inflammation of sweat glands and the formation of cysts under the arm. I would say this is reason enough not to use them.

The active ingredients in antiperspirant deodorants are aluminum compounds, which are irritants and may be absorbed into the body. We don't know the details of aluminum toxicity, but I recommend against exposing your tissues to this metal. Try natural forms of deodorants available in health food stores (the best ones contain extracts of green tea), or just splash rubbing alcohol under your arms as an antibacterial agent.

Fight Depression Without drugs?

Q:

What alternatives are there to conventional antidepressant medications or ECT (electroconvulsive or electroshock therapy)? I have tried every medical therapy possible – except ECT – but still face recurrent spontaneous episodes of major depression. Are there any alternative treatments that might short-circuit this escalating cycle?

A:

There are only two alternative treatments for depression that I have any confidence in. The first is regular aerobic exercise, which can definitely provide a long-term solution. You'll have to do at least thirty minutes of some vigorous aerobic activity at least five times a week, and be prepared to wait several weeks before you see any benefit. Aerobic exercise is a preventive as well as a treatment.

The second is an herbal treatment, called Saint-John's-wort (*Hypericum perforatum*). Saint-John's-wort is much used in Germany for the treatment of mild to moderate depression, as well as associated disturbed sleep cycles. Take 300 milligrams, three times a day, of a standardized extract containing at least 0.125 per cent hypericin. Again, be prepared to wait several months before you see the full benefit.

Changes in your diet may also make a difference. Try eating less protein and fat, and more starches, fruits, and vegetables. Experiment with the following amino acid and vitamin formula, for which you can find all the ingredients in a health food store. First thing in the morning, take 1,500 milligrams of DL-phenylalanine (DLPA, an amino acid), 100 milligrams of vitamin B-6, and 500 milligrams of vitamin C, along with a piece of fruit or a small glass of juice. Don't eat again for at least an hour. (DLPA can worsen high blood pressure, so use the formula cautiously if you have this condition, and start with a dose of 100 milligrams while monitoring your blood pressure.) Take another 100 milligrams of B-6 and more vitamin C in the evening.

You say you've taken a variety of drugs for depression. In general, I think that the new generation of antidepressants, including Prozac, and U.S. brands Zoloft and Paxil, are less toxic and more effective than medications of the past. Collectively known as SSRIs, or selective serotonin-reuptake inhibitors, they interact with the regulating mechanism for the neurotransmitter serotonin in your brain. It's best to be cautious with any of these drugs, particularly because their makers would have you believe that no one can live a normal life without them.

Make sure you aren't taking any other medications that may contribute to depression. These include antihistamines, tranquilizers, sleeping pills, and narcotics. Recreational drugs, alcohol, and coffee can also make depression worse.

You make reference to ECT – electroconvulsive or electroshock therapy. That is a last resort for the treatment of severe depression. It does work, but I hope things won't get to the point where that's your only option.

Psychiatrists tend to look at all mental problems as stemming from disordered brain chemistry; hence their emphasis on drugs. I believe that disordered moods could just as easily lead to biochemical changes in the brain, so I look elsewhere for treatments. Buddhist psychology views depression as the necessary consequence of seeking stimulation. It counsels us to cultivate emotional balance in life, rather than always seeking highs and then regretting the lows that follow. The prescription is daily meditation, and I agree this may be the best way to get at the root of depression and change it.

Doubt the Need to Douche?

Q:

My doctor says this is a growing problem among women: Advertisers try very hard to make women feel unclean so they will buy their products. Douching washes away certain forms of bacteria that protect women from getting infections. When the bacteria aren't there, a woman's body becomes more vulnerable. I'd like to hear your opinion on this.

A:

Douching used to be conventional wisdom, but it's not anymore. Now medical opinion generally discourages women from douching. And when the concern is about hygiene or odor, the risks of douching are much greater than the benefits. Douching can change the pH (or acidity level) of your vagina to be less friendly to helpful bacteria and more attractive to the harmful ones. It can wash away protective flora and leave the tissues more likely to get inflamed or infected.

In her book *Women's Bodies, Women's Wisdom*, Christiane Northrup, M.D., comments on the way women are taught to believe that the vagina is offensive, requiring deodorants and special sanitization. She says about one-third of all women douche regularly, even though it can indeed cause harm.

There are times, however, that douching can be useful in the short term. For instance, I often recommend douching with acidophilus or diluted tea tree oil for a vaginal infection. You can insert acidophilus culture directly into your vagina in capsule or liquid form. It's a 'friendly' organism that will keep overaggressive populations of yeast at bay. Tea tree oil, extracted from the leaves of the Australian tree *Melaleuca alternifolia*, is a powerful germicide. Mix about 1½ tablespoons in a cup of warm water to treat yeast infections. Some women are sensitive to this substance; discontinue it at once if you notice any irritation or burning.

Douching also may sometimes serve a protective function. Ejaculation of semen increases the pH of the vagina for eight hours. If you've had intercourse with ejaculation at least three times in a twenty-four-hour period, it will change the pH of the vagina throughout that time and produce conditions more likely for certain bacteria to grow. A douche with 1 tablespoon of white vinegar per pint and a half of warm water will help prevent problems.

Truth About
Endometriosis?

Q:
What special recommendations would you make regarding diet for endometriosis sufferers? Do you think this is an autoimmune disease?

A:
I don't know what the root cause of endometriosis is. Nobody does. It's a poorly understood disease, and the treatments are only partly helpful. The symptoms can be debilitating or just very bothersome: severe cramping, painful menstrual bleeding, intestinal gas, and sometimes depression. The condition is characterized by tissue that looks and behaves just like the lining of the uterus (endometrium), but that grows elsewhere in the body: the abdominal cavity, the intestines, the ovaries, or the abdominal wall. And just like the lining of the uterus, this tissue builds up with the hormonal changes over the month, then breaks down and bleeds. Blood in the abdomen causes intense inflammation that can be very painful. In some women, the result is severe scarring and organ dysfunction. Endometriosis also is often associated with infertility, but hasn't been shown to cause it directly.

Endometriosis doesn't necessarily progress to damage within the pelvis, or contribute to infertility. Sometimes it's very hard to find it in the body, but more and more doctors are learning that it's quite common, with as many as half of menstruating women living with it. So some experts now believe that mild endometriosis may actually be normal and not need any treatment. In fact, studies have found that in many instances it doesn't spread and grow worse over time at all.

The most popular theory about endometriosis rests on the idea that menstrual flow sometimes moves backward and up through the fallopian tubes, then out into areas within the pelvis. There the discarded tissue seems to implant and begin to grow. The hypothesis you mention is one of the most recent – that the immune system is misbehaving, failing to kill off stray endometrial cells and then pumping up their growth. Women with painful endometriosis often make antibodies against their own tissue, the hallmark of autoimmunity.

It's commonly held that pregnancy will protect against endometriosis, but recent studies have found no difference in incidence between women who have been pregnant and those who have not. It is clear that the condition is strongly affected by hormones, and hormone therapy is the favored treatment. I'd suggest minimizing your intake of estrogen from outside sources, such as commercially raised animal foods. Eat soy foods such as tofu, tempeh, and miso, which are rich in plant estrogens that can block more harmful forms of estrogen. Reduce the fat in your diet. Reduce your alcohol intake. Make sure you get nourishing food and eat lots of fiber. Exercise regularly. Also, cut dairy foods from your diet. Try all this for one month and see whether it reduces the pain.

Stress will worsen this condition. Visualization, hypnotherapy, and Chinese medicine can all be helpful. You may want to consult with an herbalist as well. Dr. Christiane Northrup has an excellent chapter on endometriosis in *Women's Bodies, Women's Wisdom*. She suggests taking a multivitamin with plenty of B-complex and magnesium (about 50 milligrams of each of the B vitamins and 400 to 800 milligrams of magnesium), in addition to maintaining a low-fat, high-fiber diet.

To Fast or Not to Fast to Lose Weight?

Q:

Is fasting an effective diet tactic? What are the best method and duration for a fast? What other sorts of health benefits or detriments are involved?

A:

Fasting is absolutely not an effective diet tool, because it will alter your metabolism in a direction that actually makes it harder to shed pounds. Most people, when they go back to eating, usually compensate by upping their consumption of calories.

There are benefits to fasting for purposes other than weight loss. (By fasting, I mean taking in nothing other than water or herbal teas. Restricting yourself to fruits, fruit juices, or other liquids can be helpful, but not in exactly the same way as fasting.) I have experimented with fasting one day a week. This can be a useful physical and psychological discipline. Many people experience a clearer mental state and increased energy after a short-term fast.

Short-term fasting for up to three days is a good home remedy for illnesses like colds, flus, and toxic conditions generally. Combine it with rest and good mental states. Drink plenty of water to help remove toxic products from your system. Also remember to conserve energy, stay warm, and break your fast with light, plain foods.

Long-term fasting – more than three days – can be beneficial but also dangerous, so do not attempt it without expert supervision. It is a drastic technique. I know some people who have fasted from one to three months and achieved complete remission of diseases that resisted all other treatments (bronchial asthma, rheumatoid arthritis, ulcerative colitis); unfortunately, the diseases often return when eating resumes.

Getting Enough
Folic Acid?

Q:

*How important is folic acid? Can't I get this and other B
vitamins in a balanced diet?*

A:

Folic acid, the synthetic form of the B vitamin folate, is
incredibly important. For one thing, folate is a key regulator of an amino acid called homocystine, a
breakdown product of animal protein. A number of
studies have connected high levels of homocystine in
the blood to arterial disease and heart attacks. Folate
helps the body eliminate homocystine from the blood.
Recently, Dr. Howard Morrison, an epidemiologist in
Ottawa, was able to make a direct connection between
folate and heart disease. He looked at folate levels in
the blood of 5,056 men who had participated in a nutrition study in the 1970s, and he found that those with
low levels of the vitamin were 69 per cent more likely to
have died from heart problems in the years since.

Folate also has been found to prevent neural tube
defects (such as spina bifida and anencephaly) in babies,
caused when this structure fails to form properly. The
neural tube is the embryonic tissue that later becomes the
brain and spinal cord. Apparently folic acid is essential to

its proper development. The U.S. Food and Drug Administration has ordered pasta, rice, and flour makers to add folic acid to their foods since January 1998 as protection against birth defects. This is partly because folic acid plays its important role in neural tube development during the first twenty-eight days of conception – usually before the woman knows she is pregnant – so it doesn't help to tell women to take vitamin supplements during pregnancy.

Folate also may be involved in preventing a whole range of chronic diseases. As the folic acid fortification rule moves into place, we may see a number of health benefits. In fact, since the Morrison study, some doctors are saying the government should double its folic acid RDA (recommended daily allowance), from 200 micrograms to 400 micrograms, to help people protect their hearts.

Folic acid is abundant in dark-green leafy vegetables, carrots, torula yeast, orange juice, asparagus, beans, and wheat germ. But as many as 90 per cent of Americans don't get that protective 400 micrograms in their diet – for example, you'd have to eat two cups of steamed spinach, a cup of boiled lentils, or eight oranges every day. So it's important to take a supplement.

A few cautions, though: Some people are allergic to the folic acid in pills. Also, anyone with a history of convulsive disorders or hormone-related cancer should not take doses above 400 micrograms a day for extended periods. Finally, high levels of folate can mask the signs of vitamin B-12 deficiency. Older people and vegetarians, who are most at risk for deficiencies in B-12, should make sure they're also getting enough of that vitamin if

Is the Fabled
G-spot for Real?

Q:
My friend and I have a disagreement over whether a woman's 'G' spot is medical fact or psychosomatic fiction. What do you think?

A:
The G-spot has not been accepted as medical fact, although many sexologists believe that it may bring about vaginal orgasm. Still, many men and women say they have located it. I even know of one feminist writer who was politically opposed to the idea of a G-spot, but who now says it's real after taking a workshop in tantric sex.

The G-spot is named after a man named Grafenberg, who first described it. If you want to experiment with finding it, the best method is for the woman to sit atop the man, facing his feet. Then you can experiment with finding the spot, which is inside the vagina between the cervix and the pubic bone. If you're flying solo, you can search for it yourself.

Another way is to study tantra, the ancient Indian art of using sexual energy to connect with the divine intimacy. Tantra workshops are now being offered around the U.S.A., but as it's being taught today, this tantra might not have any relationship to Indian tantra. One of the main techniques being taught, however, is finding the G-spot and massaging it. Proponents of modern tantra claim that women experience incredible orgasms because of this stimulation and ejaculate large volumes of fluid. The idea isn't new: ancient Chinese sexual philosophy called female ejaculation 'the tide of Yin'.

I wouldn't get too obsessed with finding a magical spot as the center for female pleasure. Anxiety and emphasis on orgasm can be the quickest route to unhappy sexual experience. Have fun exploring, and stay in touch with the intimacy and pleasure of love-making.

How Hazardous
Are Hair Dyes?

Q:
Is it safe to use hair dyes regularly?

A:
In general, I discourage people from using hair dyes.
Artificial colors are suspect in cosmetic products, just as
they are in your food. And when you apply hair dyes to
your head, they're absorbed through the scalp, where
there's a very rich blood supply that may carry them
throughout the body. There has been some speculation
that hair dyes can increase the risk of bladder cancer.
That's because the chemicals in the dye are absorbed,
and they concentrate in the bladder. Dark dyes are of
particular concern, because they contain a higher concentration of chemicals than the light ones.

I was surprised to learn that about half of all women
in the United States dye their hair – an increase of about
50 per cent in the past decade. And the hair-dye market
for middle-aged men is expected to grow rapidly –
already one in eight men between the ages of thirteen
and seventy use dyes. Commercial hair-dye makers sell
$7 billion worth of their products worldwide every year.

The most recent research on hair dyes and cancer, a

seven-year study of 573,369 women by the American Cancer Society, didn't find a significantly increased risk. Women who used very dark dyes over a period of twenty years or more did have a greater potential to develop bone cancer and non-Hodgkin's lymphoma, however. It has been suggested that dyes could have been a cause of Jacqueline Onassis's cancer. And other studies have associated an increased risk of cancer with hair dyes.

Cancer or no, dyes aren't very healthy for your hair. They can cause it to become brittle and break easily. Curiously, hair dyes aren't subject to U.S. Food and Drug Administration requirements for safety testing; they were exempted in 1938.

In general, I would stay away from chemical dyes. If you do plan to use them, make sure you don't leave the dye on your head any longer than necessary. Rinse your scalp thoroughly with water when you're done. Wear gloves during the whole process.

Henna, a plant-derived dye, is okay to use. And you can find other natural dyes in health food stores. I would stick with those.

Home Tests
for HIV?

Q:
Are over-the-counter HIV tests accurate or reliable?

A:
The U.S. Food and Drug Administration approved home HIV tests after a great deal of debate. When the first tests were submitted for regulatory scrutiny, there was much concern about accuracy. On top of that, the FDA and some AIDS activists worried that people would not get the psychological help they needed when they learned the results of positive tests. This information can be extremely upsetting. People who are tested at clinics or by their doctors always receive their results in person – from a trained professional. Counseling is critical to understanding what the results mean, learning how to cope with them, and finding out about treatment (if one is infected). Many people feel there is just no substitute for face-to-face counseling. In the U.K., all the main HIV/AIDS organizations have opposed home testing because they stress the importance of good counseling before and after the test. There are also strict regulations as to who can perform the tests, so home test kits are unlikely to be available in the U.K. in the near future.

However, in the U.S.A. the FDA ultimately decided that the tests were highly accurate and that they assured patient anonymity and provided appropriate counseling. It was thought that this option would allow more people to be tested and to know their HIV status, which in turn could stem the tide of new infections. In one survey, many people said they preferred the home test to going to a clinic. Men of color in particular said they were more likely to use a home test kit. And according to the Centers for Disease Control and Prevention in the U.S.A., 85 per cent of people tested in clinics don't get counseling with the results.

If it's more convenient and you decide you don't want to talk to someone in person, I think a home test is fine. Just make sure you do make use of the counseling available by phone.

The Confide HIV testing service, from a subsidiary of Johnson & Johnson, put out the first home kit on the market. In data submitted to regulators, the kit was 99.95 per cent accurate in identifying 3,940 samples of uninfected blood. It also correctly picked out all of the 150 samples infected with HIV, the virus that causes AIDS. In mid-1997, Johnson & Johnson pulled the Confide test from the market, claiming that only 90,000 tests had been processed during the previous year and that demand wasn't expected to grow. The FDA had also sent two warning letters to the company regarding the test, so it's not entirely clear why the product was pulled.

The standard Home Access test costs $29.95 for results by phone within seven days. The 'express' Home Access test is $49.95 for results within three days. Call (800) HIV TEST (448-8378) for more information.

Here's how the test works: You start by reading the instructions and pretest counseling booklet, which are in both Spanish and English. Then you prick your finger with a fingerstick in the kit and collect a blood sample. You drip three drops of blood onto a test card marked with a special identification number, and you mail it to a laboratory for HIV-antibody testing. Seven days later, you call a toll-free number, day or night, for the results. If the results are negative, an automated voice tells you so. If they are positive, you talk to a live person about them, what they mean, and how to get medical care.

It's very important to stay on the phone and talk to the counselor once you get the result. Realize that false positives do occur, so if you test positive, you should get tested again. The lab will do a second test by the same method, and if that one's positive, will perform a more sophisticated test called the Western blot.

If you test positive, the counselor will tell you about a number of drugs that lengthen life expectancy. You can also find out about medical, psychological, and legal services available to you.

Also, keep in mind that a negative result doesn't mean you never have to worry about HIV again. If you're sexually active in a nonmonogamous situation, or if you inject drugs, it's important to get tested regularly. There is a 'window' period of up to six months where you may be infected without the virus's showing up on a test.

And always use a condom or a dental dam to protect yourself during sexual intercourse. If you do inject drugs, use a clean needle.

Help for
Hot Flushes?

Q:
I have tried herb after herb and I stlll can't find the right combination to get rid of my hot flushes. I'm desperate. Can you help?

A:
It's interesting how medicine has transformed a natural phase in the cycle of women's bodies into a disorder. For many years, it was considered impolite to even mention the word (that's when menopause was referred to as 'the change'). Then menopause became one in a long list of imbalances attributed to women's reproductive systems, with proper intervention mandated. Advertisements and gynecologists bombard women with the same message: Menopause is a time of unhappiness, bringing moodiness, hot flushes, osteoporosis, and loss of youthful attractiveness. The 'life change' is actually a deficiency disease, the theory goes, and so only estrogen replacement therapy can restore vibrancy to women's bodies.

I'd recommend looking at this time of life in a new way. Instead of a symbol of ageing and the loss of childbearing ability, menopause can become a time to discover new energy, a freer self, and deeper wisdom within. Yes, there are discomforts associated with the changes in your body during this time. But these are signs of an opportunity to discover and claim the power of the second half of life.

During menopause, your body is adjusting to a change in hormone production. The ovaries stop releasing eggs, and it's no longer possible to get pregnant. The pituitary hormones, follicle-stimulating hormone (FSH), and luteinizing hormone (LH), which normally cycle during the month, begin to flow continuously at high levels. The ovaries slow down their output of estrogen, progesterone, and androgens. At the same time, other sites, such as the adrenal gland, the skin, and the brain, may take over hormone production. The ease of the transition depends greatly on a woman's stress level, emotional health, and nutritional status.

We rarely hear about women who have few problems with menopause, even though there are many of them. In non-Western cultures, menopause is often considered a time of strengthening and health for women. So first of all, it's important not to buy into the negative images and attitudes surrounding menopause in our culture.

Around 85 per cent of American women experience the hot flushes you mention during menopause. Not long ago, Jane Fonda described her first hot flush this way: 'When Ted and I were courting at a sound-and-light show in Athens, Greece, I had my first hot flush. It was dramatic and kind of exciting.' You may feel a great heat around your head and neck, sweat profusely, then feel chilled. Some women go through these episodes for a few months, some for years. Hot flushes have been linked to blocked energy and unused sexual potential, so women who fear they will lose their sex drive with menopause may be more bothered by them. One tactic is to work to free your sexual energy and overcome the messages you are getting about an expected loss of sex drive.

I personally recommend a menopausal formula that works well for most women. Buy capsules or tinctures of these herbs at a health food store: dong quai, a female tonic made from the root of *Angelica sinensis*; vitex, or chaste tree (*Vitex agnus-castus*), a regulator of the female reproductive system; and damiana (*Turnera diffusa*), a plant that has a reputation as a tonic and female aphrodisiac. Take two capsules of each of these every day at noon, or one dropperful of each tincture mixed in warm water once a day at noon. Keep taking the herbs until you don't experience any hot flushes, then begin to reduce the dose and try to stop altogether.

Another herb widely used for menopausal discomforts, including hot flushes, is black cohosh (*Cimifuga racemosa*), now available in the U.S.A. as a commercial product called Remifemin. Its effectiveness is supported by good scientific data.

Many women also find ginseng to be very helpful for hot flushes, especially in combination with vitamin E (800 IU a day of the natural form). Nutrition is also important. Soy products contain estrogenlike substances that may account for the low incidence of menopausal symptoms in Japanese women. And researchers have found that deep, slow breathing can reduce hot flushes to half, probably by calming the central nervous system.

Finally, there are other Chinese herbs that help to relieve hot flushes. I'd suggest you visit a practitioner of traditional Chinese medicine if you want to try them.

When to Get a Mammogram?

Q:
I'm totally confused by recent medical reports providing conflicting information about when women should go for mammograms. In your opinion, at what age should women start getting them on a regular basis?

A:
I don't blame you for your confusion. Public health authorities are at odds over this question, and the debate isn't over yet. Meanwhile, women are left in the dark on how best to take care of themselves.

The issue in question is whether women in their forties should get routine mammograms to screen for breast cancer in its earliest stages. In the U.K. women are routinely screened on the NHS every three years over the age of fifty, but the situation is different in the U.S.A. Very recently, the American Cancer Society issued new guidelines for mammograms, recommending that women in their forties have the cancer screening performed annually. Previous guidelines recommended mammograms every one to two years starting at age forty, and every year beginning at age fifty. The panel said that annual mammograms for women in their forties could save as many as 10,000 lives in the next five years.

According to Dr. Marilyn Leitch, an oncologist at the University of Texas Southwestern Medical Center, 'the current average two-year interval between mammograms may be too long in this age group and their faster-growing cancers.'

Just when a woman should begin mammography screening has been hotly debated in the U.S.A. since 1993, when the National Cancer Institute backed off its guideline that women should begin the screenings at age forty. In 1996 the issue took on new significance with the appearance of mixed data about the benefits of screening women in their forties.

In my opinion, one of the most important things to keep in mind is that the effectiveness of a mammogram as a diagnostic technique depends entirely on the experience and skill of the person who reads it. It's also my experience that mammograms do pick up tiny cancers that if left until palpable would be much more serious and life-threatening. I know several women whose lives were saved by early detection of breast cancer after a mammogram.

The downside, of course, is the amount of radiation involved. As readers know, I am opposed to needless exposure to X-ray radiation.

Got (Way Too Much) Milk?

Q:

While growing up, I was told that milk was the essential drink for staying healthy. Today, the advertisements from milk producers boast of vitamins, minerals, and, of course, calcium, calcium, calcium. In nature, milk is given to infants as a special diet to help them grow quickly. But is it healthy for adults?

A:

I think much of the information that you've received about milk as 'the essential drink' does come from the dairy industry. Dairy producers, of course, have a vested interest in seeing that as many people as possible become lifetime milk consumers.

In nature, animals drink milk only in infancy. And in many parts of the world, people react with disgust to the idea of drinking milk as adults. Milk is indeed a source of protein and calcium that some people do well on. But many adults have problems with one or more of its components.

Except among people of northwest European origin, 75 per cent of adults can't digest lactose, the sugar in milk. As they grow out of childhood, they stop making the enzyme that breaks down lactose during digestion. When lactose-intolerant people drink milk, they experience digestive upsets such as wind, cramps, or diarrhea.

Butterfat, the fat in milk, is the most saturated fat in the American diet. Cheese, for example, is often 70 per cent – or more – fat by calories. Milk fat is a principal contributor to high cholesterol and artery-clogging atherosclerosis.

The protein in milk, called casein, irritates many people's immune systems. This is also the component of milk that stimulates mucus production. Milk often worsens such conditions as recurrent ear infections in early life, eczema, chronic bronchitis, asthma, and sinus conditions.

Most commercial milk also contains residues from drugs, hormones, and chemicals used to keep modern dairy cows producing abundantly.

I think most people should limit their intake of whole milk and the products made from it. Lactose-intolerant adults can eat cultured milk products (such as yogurt) now and then. Nonfat yogurt, mozzarella, or other lowfat cheeses are good ways to enjoy milk products occasionally without exposing yourself to so much fat.

The dairy industry has done a great job convincing us that children are deprived without milk. I've kept my own five-year-old daughter off cow's milk. She has been remarkably healthy and has never had an ear infection.

I give her goat's milk, Rice Dream (a brown-rice beverage that comes in different flavours), or a new product in the U.S.A. called Vance's DariFree. It's made from potatoes, and I think it's the best-tasting of the milk substitutes. You should be aware that rice and potato drinks aren't protein-based. If you give any of these milk substitutes to your children, they'll need a different source of protein. (Soy milk does contain protein and is a good substitute for many people, but children are sometimes allergic to it.)

As for calcium, which helps regulate the nerves and muscles and is necessary for building strong bones, there are other ways to get it. Cooked greens (especially kales), molasses, sesame seeds, broccoli, and tofu are good sources. In adults, dairy products can do more harm than good, because their protein content can accelerate the loss of calcium from bones.

Abnormal
Pap Smear?

Q:
Can an abnormal Pap smear be an indicator for any sexually transmitted diseases? And, related to that, why is it necessary to wait four months before going back to get another Pap smear?

A:
The aim of a Pap smear, named after Dr. George Papanicolaou, is to detect abnormal cells in the cervix, the doughnut-shaped entrance to the uterus. The idea is to identify cellular changes that can lead to cancer before they get out of control. The procedure is simple: a gynecologist or trained nurse uses a soft brush, called a cytobrush, or a small wooden or plastic spatula to sample cells from just inside the cervical opening and from the outside. The cells are fixed on a slide and sent to a laboratory for analysis.

The Pap smear itself is not a diagnostic test for sexually transmitted diseases, but it can reveal conditions associated with them. In fact, most abnormal Pap slides result from infection with the human papillomavirus (HPV), not any malignancy. HPV is a very common sexually transmitted infection that causes venereal warts and is associated with cervical cancer. It's believed that you have to have HPV in order to develop cancer of the cervix. But HPV doesn't automatically lead to cancer – it just means you should be extra vigilant and get Pap smears yearly.

Most cervical cell changes discovered through a Pap smear return to normal on their own within a few months. That's why gynecologists will usually wait four months, then repeat the test. If the second test comes back clear, then it's best to repeat the smear a third time to make sure you get two negative tests in a row. False negatives occur often enough that I wouldn't be satisfied with just one negative result.

Cervical cancer is slow-growing, so a wait of four months shouldn't be a problem. If you want to be extra careful, or the second test comes back positive, you can have the abnormal tissue removed right away.

You should also know the risk factors for cervical cancer. These include infection with HPV, multiple childbirths, smoking, multiple sexual partners, first intercourse before age sixteen, and having a suppressed immune system. Whether or not any of these apply, however, I'd still recommend a Pap test once a year. In the U.K. the NHS routinely screens women once every three years until the age of fifty, then once every five years (more often if you have any abnormality). The symptoms of cervical cancer include bleeding between periods or after intercourse, and abnormal vaginal discharge.

Women with cervical abnormalities tend to have weakened immune systems. They may suffer from low levels of vitamin A, B-complex vitamins – especially folic acid – and antioxidants. They may be experiencing extra stress. To help protect yourself against cellular changes in the cervix, the best thing to do is take good care of yourself and take my antioxidant cocktail (see page 3), plus a B-complex supplement that provides 400 micrograms of folic acid.

Let's Get a
Physical?

Q:
What would you recommend be included in an annual physical examination for a healthy forty-two-year-old woman? I've been trying to find information on this, but have been having trouble doing so.

A:
I'm not really a believer in general physicals every year, but if you've never had a physical exam or haven't had one in a long while, it's worth getting one done. Healthy women in their twenties and thirties don't have to worry much about annual exams, but it would be a good idea to get one at some point as a baseline to compare with later. (In the U.K. a comprehensive physical would not be available on the NHS, but it is possible to have one privately.) General physicals become important as you enter your forties and fifties; then it makes sense to think about doing exams on a more regular basis.

The procedure should include both a history – your answers to questions about past illnesses and present symptoms – and a physical examination by a doctor. It's important that you talk to your doctor about anything that troubles you about your health. You might want to bring a list of problems and questions. (In addition to physical health, you should talk to your doctor about any emotional or psychological difficulties.) Remember, most doctors are working under factory-like conditions these days, and you've got to make sure you get the attention you're there for. Be an assertive patient.

There are standard items that should be included in the physical part of the exam. There may be other tests, depending on your medical history. Usually the doctor will start with pulse and blood pressure and a check of your heart, lungs, and lymph nodes.

For anyone in his or her forties, the visit should include a rectal examination, plus a stool sample to test for blood. For women, the exam should also include a vaginal examination and a Pap smear. Women should go every two years for a Pap smear (to check for cancer of tbe cervix), a breast exam, and a pelvic exam.

There is also a standard panel of blood tests (SMAC 20) that should be done, as well as a complete blood count. I would also include a complete lipid panel to determine cholesterol and other blood fats. Your urine should be sampled for testing, too.

Women should have a mammogram by at least age fifty, and possibly a baseline one earlier. You might think about it earlier if you have a family history of breast cancer or any reason to think you're at higher risk. New guidelines recommend annual mammograms beginning at age forty (see page 41).

Eyeing Plastic Surgery?

Q:

I am thinking about having cosmetic surgery on my eyelids. I am only in my late twenties, but I have to do it because my eyelids really drag down. I don't know what I will look like afterward; all I can imagine is how horrific I am going to look with the stitches in. I believe there is a lot of bruising. I know that if I could see some pictures of what other people look like after surgery it would put my mind at ease. I have asked the plastic surgeon for some pictures, but he says he doesn't have any. (I am afraid he might also think I am a real chicken if I persist with this query.) What can I do about this anxiety, and the shock I will get when I see my eyes like that?

A:

First, please don't agree to have cosmetic surgery without really thinking it through carefully – not just about what it may look like along the way and afterward, but also about what you expect from it and why you want it. Be sure you really want this surgery. Ask your surgeon to explain in detail all the things that can go wrong. Find out what results the surgery can and can't produce. If your surgeon can't or won't tell you, find a different surgeon. I've written before about the importance of being an assertive patient; that remains important when you are considering elective surgery. In the U.S.A., the cost for upper and lower lids can be as much as $7,000.

As for your immediate concerns, you're right: you have to be prepared for the week or two after surgery when you'll look worse than you did when you went in. And it takes from five to eight weeks until you're completely healed. A good resource for anyone considering plastic surgery is Diana Barry's *Nips & Tucks: Everything You Must Know before Having Cosmetic Surgery*. Barry covers everything from eyelid surgery to collagen injections to postmastectomy reconstruction.

Other, more invasive surgeries – like face-lifts – can take quite a bit more time to heal fully (and there can be some permanent side effects). I've seen some very good results from cosmetic surgery. But I've also seen a number of cases where people's faces ended up looking very unnatural to me. The skin can look stretched and too tight. You really need to make sure you're working with a very good cosmetic surgeon who can clearly explain what the result of the surgery will look like.

I don't know if you smoke, but be aware that people who smoke tobacco are at higher risk for complications from cosmetic surgery, because they have decreased blood circulation in the skin. Smoking can also impair and delay healing. If you can't quit altogether, your surgeon will suggest stopping ten days before surgery, and for a week post-op. That's the minimum.

I also have to say that all this sounds highly premature. You said you're in your twenties, which is very young to be considering cosmetic surgery. Ask yourself a few basic questions before you do anything else. Why aren't you happy with yourself as you are? Is your unhappiness with your eyelids reflective of a larger kind of dissatisfaction with your being? Does your decision to change your eyelids rest on what other people have been telling you about your appearance? Maybe there are other ways you can become happier without having to undergo surgery. You may want to talk over the possibilities with a therapist before going any further.

SOS for PMS?

Q:

I am a victim of premenstrual syndrome (PMS). It has become progressively worse in the past year, I'd say. My moods are so extreme, it is difficult for me to be around other humans. I go from being filled with rage and hostility to feeling anxious and scared for no reason, to sobbing uncontrollably at the drop of a hat. I recently went on the Pill, which has made my cycle more predictable, but I'm still an emotional basket case. My boyfriend is ready to kill me. Please help.

A:

Many male doctors consider PMS an imaginary condition, and some feminists believe it's a construct of the male establishment. Nevertheless, many women suffer severe physical discomfort, plus the mood swings you mention, just before the onset of menstruation. Common symptoms include depression, tension, anger, difficulty concentrating, lethargy, changes in appetite, and a feeling of being overwhelmed. These can be accompanied by breast tenderness, headache, fluid retention, and joint or muscle pain. PMS's effects may begin around the time of ovulation, then diminish during menstruation or just after.

It is possible to ease the severity of PMS or even eliminate it entirely. First, I'd suggest removing all caffeine – including chocolate – from your life. Many women crave chocolate just before menstruation and say it acts as an antidepressant. But it can be addictive and can have a powerful effect on moods, energy cycles, and sleep patterns. Caffeine adds to nervous tension and increases your heart rate. (So beware of using caffeine or chocolate as a spiritual or emotional salve.) Also avoid all polyunsaturated vegetable oils, which can promote inflammation.

Next, you should exercise regularly. I would suggest twenty to thirty minutes of some sustained aerobic activity five days a week. Besides giving a sense of strength and well-being, and increasing the flow of oxygen to all organs, exercise helps to regulate your hormone levels.

Third, take a supplement of evening primrose oil or black currant oil, two capsules two or three times a day. Both supplements supply an unusual fatty acid called gamma-linolenic acid (GLA), an effective anti-inflammatory agent. (GLA also promotes healthy skin, hair, and nails.) Try this for at least two months and continue if you feel better. I would also take supplements of calcium and magnesium, preferably 1,200 to 1,500 milligrams of calcium citrate at bedtime, and half that amount of magnesium. These may ease menstrual cramps.

You might experiment with several herbs that have a good track record with PMS. The first is dong quai, a

Chinese remedy made from the root of *Angelica sinensis* in the carrot family. It acts as a general tonic for the female reproductive system in much the same way that ginseng works for men. You can try two capsules twice a day for several months to see how it affects you. Another possibility is vitex, or chaste tree (*Vitex agnus-castus*), in the same dosage. It helps regulate the female reproductive cycle. Try these one at a time to assess their benefit. (See also page 81, for a sedative tea.)

As a general tonic for your mind, body, and moods, experiment with deep breathing and other relaxation techniques. It also may be helpful to analyze which symptoms you are feeling and when. Try listing the symptoms that bother you most, then recording when you experience them during the month. This can help you be aware of what to expect each month, and also clarify which symptoms are actually tied to your menstrual cycle and which might have another cause.

Smoking Pot
While Pregnant?

Q:
Has there been any research that suggests the effects of marijuana use during pregnancy?

A:
In general, it is wise to avoid putting any drugs into your body during the first three months of pregnancy, when most fetal development is taking place. It makes sense to take as few drugs as possible during the rest of the pregnancy as well.

Of the common recreational drugs in use, however, marijuana is probably less risky than nicotine, alcohol, and even caffeine. Coffee, for example, may increase the risk of miscarriage. Alcohol increases the probability of birth defects. Mothers who smoke cigarettes have more miscarriages and often give birth to babies with below-normal birth weights.

Marijuana is a less powerful pharmacological agent, so the adverse effects are likely to be less severe, although there is little evidence documenting them. One study reported in *The New England Journal of Medicine* in 1989 did associate marijuana use with impaired fetal growth.

The bottom line: Don't put foreign substances into your body during pregnancy, especially during the first three months. Smoking (marijuana or cigarettes) around the baby is also not a good idea, since babies are very sensitive to smoke of all kinds.

Commit to Quit Smoking?

Q:

I know I should quit. I just can't seem to. I desperately need help.

A:

I know that many smokers stare at themselves in the mirror, asking, 'How do I quit?' It's hard. Tobacco, in the form of cigarettes, is the most addictive drug in the world – and that says a lot. There are two reasons for this: Nicotine is one of the strongest stimulants known, and smoking is one of the most efficient drug-delivery systems. Smoking actually puts drugs into the brain more directly than intravenous injection.

In the early part of this century, cigarette smoking was accepted, and was even considered healthy and glamorous. It was seen as a way to promote mental acuity, efficiency, and relaxation. It is true that one of the 'benefits' of smoking is brief relief of internal tension; unfortunately, within twenty minutes tension returns, requiring another fix.

Low-tar, low-nicotine cigarettes offer no great advantages. People tend to smoke more of them, or inhale more deeply to get the same amount of nicotine. Pipes and cigars, if the smoke is not inhaled, do not cause lung cancer and emphysema, but they do increase the risk of oral cancer (as do snuff and chewing tobacco).

I feel so strongly about people not smoking that I will not accept patients who are users unless they have made a commitment to try to quit. There are many programs available to help you do so: acupuncture, hypnotherapy, and support groups. There are also a slew of new devices – nicotine patches and gum, for instance – on the market that work for some. None of these methods works reliably for everyone. Most successful quitters do it on their own after one or more unsuccessful attempts. Going 'cold turkey' also seems to work better than gradually cutting down.

Don't get discouraged. If you can't quit today, you may be able to tomorrow. You want to be motivated. You need to do this for yourself, not because someone else wants you to. Remember: You get credit for every attempt you make. In fact, the best predictor for success is making attempts to quit.

If you smoke, do this breathing exercise. It will help motivate you to quit and help you with your cravings for cigarettes. Here's how to start.

1. Sit with your back straight. Place the tip of your tongue against the ridge of tissue behind your upper front teeth, and keep it there throughout the exercise.
2. Exhale completely though your mouth, making a *whoosh* sound.
3. Close your mouth and inhale quietly through your nose to a mental count of four.
4. Hold your breath for a count of seven.

5. Exhale completely through your mouth, again making a *whoosh* sound, to a count of eight.
6. This is one breath. Now inhale again and repeat the cycle three more times.

If you smoke, you should take antioxidant vitamins and minerals (see page 3), which to some extent can reverse the changes in respiratory tissue caused by smoking, and so help protect against lung cancer. Also, increase your intake of dietary sources of carotenes: carrots, sweet potatoes, yellow squash, and leafy green vegetables).

Good luck, and please set a date for your next attempt to quit.

Weight Loss with Redux?

Q:
I have been taking Redux for about one month now, with mixed results. The first two weeks I completely lost my appetite (which wasn't so bad, as I was 360 pounds), and I would only remember to eat when I got weak. Is this common? What's the word on Redux? Also, I've noticed a complete lack of depressive episodes, which I get chronically. Is this due to the fact that Redux is a serotonin-reuptake inhibitor? Thanks.

A:
Redux, which last year became the first new diet drug to be approved by U.S. federal regulators in twenty-three years, has been embraced wholeheartedly by dieters and diet clinics, and is expected to become a $1 million drug during its first five years. But the Food and Drug Administration in the U.S.A. has some reservations about its safety, and physicians are worried about its overuse.

While Redux has promise for some people, it certainly is not the answer to obesity. Maybe sometime in the future we will fine-tune these pharmacological approaches. But at the moment, Redux and all the others remain fairly crude drugs, even though they're better than drugs we've had in the past.

Redux is indicated chiefly for people who are very overweight, rather than moderately overweight. Some of the more common side effects include fatigue, diarrhea, vivid dreams, and dry mouth. There are also some serious, albeit rare, toxic effects; you wouldn't want to risk these unless you really needed help with health-threatening weight problems.

Redux works by stimulating the serotonin system in the brain, thus making people feel satisfied and full. It certainly could produce the alleviation of depression you're enjoying. In fact, some scientists think it's actually the mood elevation you're feeling that helps you stop eating and lose weight. An older diet drug, fenfluramine, which is taken in combination with phentermine, was developed on this principle. Researchers found that high levels of carbohydrates in the blood boosted serotonin levels, which then improved mood. They theorized that people may overeat high-carbohydrate foods in an effort to boost their mood. Fenfluramine, like Redux, boosts serotonin production, overriding a person's drive to overeat.

This all sounds great, but there are problems with artificially boosting serotonin. Redux has caused brain damage in rats and monkeys. In slight overdose, the drug apparently causes the neurons that make serotonin in the brain to burn out. Some of the neurons regenerate, but usually without hooking up to the right connections. Long-term results could include memory loss, depression, concentration problems, and sleep disturbances. Redux also raises the risk of pulmonary hypertension, a potentially fatal disorder that tightens up blood vessels in the lungs to the point where the heart may fail while trying to pump blood through them.

Another problem with any drug like Redux involves getting off it once you've lost the weight you want. With most pharmacological weight-loss treatments, the pounds come right back once you stop taking the drugs. So you can't use Redux alone. You have to add a regular program of exercise to your life, and change your eating habits. It's simple, but not always easy: you must eat less and exercise more. Also keep in mind that the more gradually you lose the weight, the more likely it is you will maintain your slimmer self.

What's Up with RU-486 (the Abortion Pill)?

Q:
Was RU-486 approved, and where is it available?

A:
RU-486, the French abortion pill, is still making its way through an obstacle course into the U.S. drug system – although it's now very close to approval. The Food and Drug Administration recently said it would allow sale of the drug, pending more information on how RU-486 will be labeled and manufactured. There will be certain rules to ensure its safety. For example, doctors who prescribe it must meet certain requirements, and women who take it must live within an hour of emergency treatment in case something goes wrong.

I'm happy to see this drug finally become available as an option for women who want abortions. Known chemically as mifepristone, it's vastly superior to the methods available now. Still, RU-486 should not be taken lightly. It requires three steps. First, the woman takes 600 milligrams of RU-486 to end the pregnancy. It's 95.5 per cent effective when used within the first seven weeks. Then she must take another drug to induce contractions in the uterus to expel the fetus.

Finally, she must go back in for an exam to make sure the pregnancy has been aborted.

Using this drug is much less traumatic than undergoing surgery. The side effects are similar to those of a spontaneous miscarriage: bleeding, cramps, nausea, and fatigue. Serious complications are rare. In clinical trials in the United States, 4 out of 2,100 women needed a blood transfusion because of uncontrolled bleeding.

Women began using RU-486 in France in 1988. Protests by antiabortion groups were so venomous, however, that manufacturer Roussel-Uclaf suspended distribution. Almost immediately, the French Minister of Health stepped forward and ordered the company to sell the drug in the interest of public health. I've heard that about 200,000 women have used the drug in Europe – it's approved in France, the United Kingdom (where it is known as Mifegyne), and Sweden. In the United States, the Bush administration was not so open-minded. It banned the import of RU-486. Clinton lifted the prohibition in 1993, and Roussel-Uclaf gave the rights for the drug to a nonprofit research institution in New York, the Population Council, which began clinical trials here to test safety and effectiveness.

An FDA advisory committee recommended approval for RU-486 in July 1996; then the FDA announced in September 1996 that it was ready to approve the drug, which will probably be renamed in the United States.

A Proven Sex-Drive
Enhancer?

Q:
Is there anything I can take to boost my sex drive? I'm female.

A:
Of course, people have been asking this question for centuries. Curiously enough, a proven sex-drive enhancer for women is the male hormone testosterone. Women produce their own testosterone, and reputable scientific studies show that tiny additional amounts can increase libido dramatically. One testosterone product, formulated in the U.S.A. for women in menopause, is called Estratest (unavailable in the U.K.); it also contains estrogen.

An herbal possibility for women is the Mexican plant damiana (*Turnera diffusa*), which has a reputation as a female aphrodisiac. Not that much is known about it, but you can find damiana preparations in health food stores. Again, follow dosage recommendations on the label. Whichever of these appeals to you, try it for a few months and see what it can do for you. If it works, great. If not, there's no point in continuing the treatment.

But before spending money on substances like these, you might want to consider other ways to boost sexual energy. Both physical and mental well-being are important to healthy sex. Think about the interplay of emotional charge, mental imagery, and body responses associated with sex. Hypnotherapy and guided imagery therapy can help you make the most of the mind-body connection in overcoming sexual problems. Many experts, myself included, say the greatest aphrodisiac is the human mind.

Dangers of Silicone Implants?

Q:

I have never heard you speak on what women who have breast implants can do to help rid their bodies of the silicone gel. Many of us have developed multiple problems and are in a daily search for help. Any and all information would be greatly appreciated and shared with many.

A:

Women with side effects from breast implants often get hopeless prognoses from doctors, or else get treated as if their problems were imaginary. Medical literature does not support the existence of silicone disease, but it is obvious to me that women who have had silicone in their bodies may suffer from a variety of autoimmune reactions. In the U.S.A., the Food and Drug Administration put a halt to silicone implants in 1992 because of concerns about their safety.

I don't think it's a great idea to have silicone in the body, so if you've experienced any problems, I'd recommend having the breast implants removed. It's a tougher question if you're not having problems. If the implants are undamaged and intact, you're probably okay – and it may not be worth the trauma to have them removed. On the other hand, the implants can develop slow leaks, with complications showing up later. One sign of a problem is your breast becoming hard. An FDA panel estimated in 1992 that up to 6 per cent of silicone implants rupture. If you're unsure – or just concerned – about the status of your implants, talk to your doctor; he or she can detect abnormalities by ultrasound mammography.

I don't know of any way to remove the silicone that may have leaked into your tissues. But I have seen great improvement in women who had the implants removed and then followed a program to improve their general health.

If you're experiencing problems, here are some steps you should take:

- Eat a low-protein diet, eliminate milk and milk products, and cut back on meat and other foods of animal origin.
- Avoid polyunsaturated oils.
- Eat fish and organically grown fruits, vegetables, and grains.
- Take antioxidant vitamins and minerals.
- Exercise regularly.
- Practise relaxation techniques and experiment with visualization, psychotherapy, and hypnotherapy.
- Consider traditional Chinese medical treatment or Ayurvedic medicine.
- Try ginger, which has an anti-inflammatory effect, as do feverfew and turmeric.

If you're experiencing autoimmune arthritis, I

recommend one to two capsules of powdered, dried ginger twice a day, or one to two capsules of freeze-dried feverfew leaves twice a day. You can take turmeric in the form of curcumin (the active component, which happens to give turmeric its yellow pigment) in 400- to 600-milligram doses three times a day.

Could It Be
Skin Cancer?

Q:
I've had a small, scab-like sore on my thigh for fifteen to twenty years. I suspect skin cancer. Is it really dangerous to ignore it? How fast does skin cancer grow, and how does it grow?

A:
Skin cancers are the most common form of cancer, and their incidence is climbing dramatically. The number of cases of melanoma – the deadliest form of skin cancer – alone grew by 21 per cent in the past decade.

People are also getting better at spotting skin cancer, and that's very good news, because early treatment cures 95 per cent of people with the disease. That's why it's important to pay attention to the kind of sore you've described.

Any sore that doesn't heal should be examined by a dermatologist. And even though you've had this one for such a long time, it's possible that it may have changed without your noticing. There's really no hard-and-fast rule for how quickly skin cancers grow. Some grow very slowly; others don't. In general, a sore that doesn't heal is a cause for concern. Only a medical professional can tell you what to do about it.

When checking yourself for signs of skin cancer, you should look for changes in freckles or moles and any new bumps or nodules. Are any moles larger than the diameter of a pencil eraser? Are they of mixed colors (especially including black)? Are their borders irregular? Do the areas around them look inflamed or pale? Are they getting bigger? Are they scaly, scabby, or do they fail to heal after a minor injury? If you answer yes to any of these questions, it doesn't necessarily mean the moles or other areas are cancerous, but it does mean they deserve examination.

The risk of melanoma is particularly high in people who have family histories of the disease, and in those who've experienced blistering sunburns before age twenty. Everyone should wear sunscreen every day (SPF-15, at least), cover up with long-sleeve, tight-weave clothing, and stay indoors or in the shade when the sun is highest in the sky and in the months around the summer solstice.

If you start taking these kinds of precautions now, you can dramatically reduce the chance of developing skin cancer later in life.

How's Now
with the Tao?

Q:

What are your impressions of the Chinese Tao of sex? Claims are that by withholding ejaculation the body is strengthened, the mind made clearer, vision and hearing are improved, and the man feels closer to and more loving toward his mate. As reluctant as I may be to accept the concept completely, my limited experience with the Taoist approach seems to indicate more truth than fiction. Any comments?

A:

It is a widespread folk belief, especially in east Asia, that withholding semen improves mental and physical health. In ancient Chinese sexology, reserving semen was believed to prolong life and maybe lead to immortality. Something of the same belief is part of the mythology of modern sports, too. ('Don't have sex before the big game.') I don't know that there's any evidence to support the idea that infrequent ejaculation preserves health, however, or if anyone has ever done research to find out.

In thinking about the Tao of love, I think it's best not to become preoccupied with ejaculation. Over the years, the ancient Chinese theories about sex have become distorted to the point where they make sex seem like a war between men and women, in which men may seriously harm themselves by sacrificing their semen. Semen becomes a symbol of male power and life force that females covet, like vampires who suck the blood of their prey.

That's not what the Tao of love should be about. If a man can let go of the desire to ejaculate, he can relax and enjoy the peaks and valleys of lovemaking longer. Instead of thinking in terms of reaching a goal, he can concentrate on the ecstasy of touching his lover, and his lover's responses. There is time to savor each other's texture, scent, and movements.

For a woman, it's the same. Instead of striving toward orgasm, she can enjoy the pleasures of touching, caressing, and kissing. The techniques of Taoist sex reflect one underlying purpose: Rather than letting sexual energy control us, men and women should learn to control it with conscious intent. Since an ejaculation necessitates a temporary end to lovemaking, if a man can learn to enjoy the experience in other ways, the night can be very long, and very pleasurable.

For an understanding of the Taoist philosophy, I recommend two books by Jolan Chang: *The Tao of Love and Sex* and *The Tao of the Loving Couple*.

Walking for
Your Life?

Q:
*Is it true that walking is almost equal to jogging as an
aerobic exercise?*

A:
I'm a great proponent of walking. Not only is it almost
equal to jogging in terms of getting your heart pumping,
but I think research will eventually show that it's superior in terms of overall health benefits. There are lots
of reasons to prefer walking to just about any other form
of exercise. First of all, everyone knows how to do it and
it doesn't require any equipment. Second, you can do it
anywhere. Third, the risk of injury is far less than for
any other kind of aerobic exercise.

With jogging, the risk of injury is high. A person who
jogs is also more likely to become exercise-dependent or
to misuse exercise. People who really go for the endor-
phin high are often tempted to run through the pain –
and then wind up being unable to exercise at all.

I will often take a walk in the morning after I medi-
tate. Or sometimes, in the afternoon, I walk around the
ranch where I live. If I'm in a city like New York or San
Francisco, I try to do as much walking as possible.

Obviously, San Francisco is great for walking because of the hills. In New York walking is wonderful because the people-watching is so interesting.

You may also find that walking can be meditative and relaxing. You can take in the sights or listen to something on a Walkman. Walking exercises your brain as well as your body; it's a cross-patterned movement (right arm moves forward with the left leg) that generates harmonizing electrical activity in your central nervous system.

I find that good running shoes with cushioned soles are best for walking. But experiment – find out what works for you. If you walk up a long, gradual hill or walk at a good clip, you can get your heart and respiratory rate high enough for the aerobic benefit. Maintain a good posture and be sure to swing your arms as you go. I recommend forty-five minutes a day, every day if possible. That's about three miles. If you can't make time to walk every day, do it at least five times a week.

What's the Perfect Workout?

Q:

How many calories should you be burning during an average workout? I tend to do half an hour of cardiovascular exercise three times a week plus occasional weight training. According to the machines, I burn 250 calories. I'm five feet four and weigh 125 pounds. Is this the right amount of exercise and calorie-burning for me?

A:

Aerobic exercise is the kind that increases your heart rate and makes you huff and puff. It promotes general fitness, conditions your heart and respiratory system, and increases stamina. It also tones your nervous and immune systems, reduces stress, increases the flow of oxygen throughout the body, and gives you a sense of strength and well-being.

For optimum cardiovascular fitness, I recommend exercising every day. Aim toward at least thirty minutes five times a week. It need not be in one continuous session. Ideally, your daily routine should also include plenty of aerobic activity, such as brisk walking, housework, gardening, and so on.

I am a great proponent of walking for fitness.

Sustained walking – especially uphill walking and brisk walking – can give a better overall workout than running or exercising intensely on aerobic machines. Walking has the advantages of not requiring any equipment and carrying the least risk of injury of any aerobic exercise. Use good posture, swing your arms, and keep a good pace. Three miles should take about forty-five minutes. I recommend running shoes for this activity – ones with well-cushioned insoles.

Specific forms of exercise have their own benefits. Swimming is great for the joints, a balanced muscular workout, and relaxation. Cycling builds knee muscles and can provide a feeling of exhilaration. Dancing is one of the best aerobic activities of all, because it's fun, never boring, and it provides a thorough workout.

Once you have developed good habits of regular exercise, you can add stretching, muscle toning, and strengthening to your routine. Yoga is a great way to stretch, improve flexibility, and experience deep relaxation. Breathing exercises, meditation, and other forms of relaxation are important to help neutralize stress.

Personally, I walk whenever possible. I use a Stair-Master occasionally, and go mountain biking in the desert. I also swim and do some weight training – and mix all of these up.

I don't think that calorie-burning is the best guide to how much exercise you should do. If your weight is stable, think in terms of overall cardiovascular fitness, strength, and flexibility. Vary your workout to keep it interesting. And, above all, have fun.

Yams for Hormone Therapy?

Q:
What's the scoop on wild yam cream? Is it merely a marketing phenomenon? Or does it have real botanical benefits for PMS sufferers and menopausal discomfort relief-seekers?

A:
Wild yam, or *Dioscorea*, is the tuber of a tropical plant. Don't expect to find it in your grocery store – it's completely unrelated to the sweet potatoes that many people call yams in this country. All sorts of claims have been made about wild yam because it contains a precursor of steroid hormones called diosgenin, which was used as the starting material for the first birth control pill. But diosgenin itself has no hormonal activity. Nor can the human body convert it into something that does.

That's why I question the efficacy of creams that contain only wild yam as the supposed source of natural hormonal activity. Some of these creams may contain synthetic progesterone, even though this doesn't show up on the label. That would certainly make them active.

Wild yam may have sedative properties that can help relieve premenstrual problems. In *Herbs for Health and*

Healing, Kathi Keville recommends a tea made of 1 teaspoon vitex berries, 1 teaspoon wild yam, ½ teaspoon each of burdock root, dandelion root, feverfew leaves, and the flowering parts of hops. Place the herbs in a pot containing a pint and a half of water and bring to a boil. Then steep for at least twenty minutes with the heat off. It may help with the cramps, emotional changes, and nausea you sometimes feel before your menstrual period. You can also buy a tincture with these herbs.

Natural Help for
Yeast Infections?

Q:
What do I do about recurring yeast infections? I've had them for over twenty years.

A:
Many women suffer from frequent vaginal yeast infections, which can indicate an underlying metabolic imbalance. It often helps if you change your diet to make your body a less appealing host for the organism. Your partner may want to do the same. (Studies suggest that treating the patient's sexual partner may stop recurrence.)

First, try reducing your sugar intake. High-sugar diets stimulate the growth of yeast. Also, add garlic to your diet. A clove once a day is a powerful natural medicine, with specific anti-yeast effects. (That's one segment from a bulb, not the whole thing!) Mash or chop it fine, mix it with food, and eat it with a meal. Or cut it into chunks and swallow the chunks like pills. Fresh-grown garlic is much better than any garlic supplements. Chew a little parsley afterward if you're concerned about odor, but if you eat garlic regularly and have a good attitude about it, you won't smell of it. Try it; it really works.

Finally, take acidophilus culture. These bacteria are the ones that make milk sour. 'Friendly' and natural to the intestinal tract, they may also out-compete yeast in the vaginal area and change the chemistry of the tissues to make them resistant to the fungi. You can buy acidophilus in health food stores, in capsules, or in a milk or carrot-juice base. Check the expiration date to make sure the bacteria are healthy. Take one tablespoon of the liquid culture or one to two of the dry capsules after meals, unless the label directs otherwise.

These changes to your diet may help reverse some of your underlying susceptibility to yeast infections. To treat the infections when they occur, try placing a capsule of acidophilus directly into your vagina once a day, or use a rubber bulb syringe to insert one tablespoon of liquid culture. Another possibility would be tea tree oil, a nontoxic treatment very useful for fungal infections. The oil is extracted from the leaves of *Melaleuca alternifolia*. You can find it in health food or herb stores. Mix 1½ tablespoons of the oil in a cup of warm water and use it as a douche once a day. If you experience any irritation, however, discontinue its use.

Resources

Books by Andrew Weil, M.D.

8 Weeks to Optimum Health: A Proven Program for Taking Full Advantage of Your Body's Natural Healing Power. London: Little, Brown, 1997.

Spontaneous Healing: How to Discover and Enhance Your Body's Natural Ability to Maintain and Heal Itself. London: Little, Brown, 1995.

Natural Health, Natural Medicine: A Comprehensive Manual for Wellness and Self-Care. Rev. ed. London: Little, Brown, 1997.

Health and Healing: Understanding Conventional and Alternative Medicine. Rev. ed. Boston: Houghton Mifflin, 1995.

From Chocolate to Morphine: Everything You Need to Know About Mind-Altering Drugs, with Winifred Rosen. Rev. ed. Boston: Houghton Mifflin, 1993.

The Natural Mind: An Investigation of Drugs and the Higher Consciousness. Rev. ed. Boston: Houghton Mifflin, 1986.

The Marriage of the Sun and the Moon: A Quest for Unity in Consciousness. Boston: Houghton Mifflin, 1980.

Other Recommended Books

Barry, Diana. *Nips & Tucks: Everything You Must Know before Having Cosmetic Surgery*. Los Angeles: General Publishing Group, 1996.

Chang, Jolan. *The Tao of Love and Sex: The Ancient Chinese Way to Ecstasy*. Aldershot: Wildwood house, 1976.

Chang, Jolan. *The Tao of the Loving Couple*. New York: Dutton, 1995.

Keville, Kathi, with Peter Korn. *Herbs for Health and Healing: The Illustrated Encyclopedia of Herbs*. Emmaus, Pennsylvania: Rodale Press, 1996.

Northrup, Christiane, M.D. *Women's Bodies, Women's Wisdom: Creating Physical and Emotional Health and Healing*. New York: Bantam Books, 1995.

Other Resources

Foresight (preconceptual care)
28 The Paddock
Godalming
Surrey
Tel: 01483 427839

Health Education Authority
Trevelyan House
30 Great Peter Street
London SW1P 2HW
Tel: 0171 222 5300

National Childbirth Trust
Alexandra House
Oldham Terrace
London W3 6NH
Tel: 0181 992 8637
For local branches see your telephone directory.

Soil Association
Bristol House
40–56 Victoria Street
Bristol
BS1 6BY
Tel: 0117 929 0661

Program in Integrative Medicine

At the University of Arizona Health Sciences Center, Tucson, Arizona. For more information, visit the Web site: http://www.ahsc.arizona.edu/integrative_medicine. Or write: Center for Integrative Medicine, P.O. Box 64089, Tucson, AZ 85718.

Newsletter
If you would like information on my lectures and informational products, including my monthly newsletter, *Self Healing*, please write to: Andrew Weil, M.D., P.O. Box 457, Vail, AZ 85641.

On the Web
'Ask Dr. Weil' answers health questions daily on Time Warner's Pathfinder Network (www.drweil.com).

Index

Acknowledgments

Richard Pine, Judith Curr, Elisa Wares, and Scott Fagan.